Plant based cook book for beginners

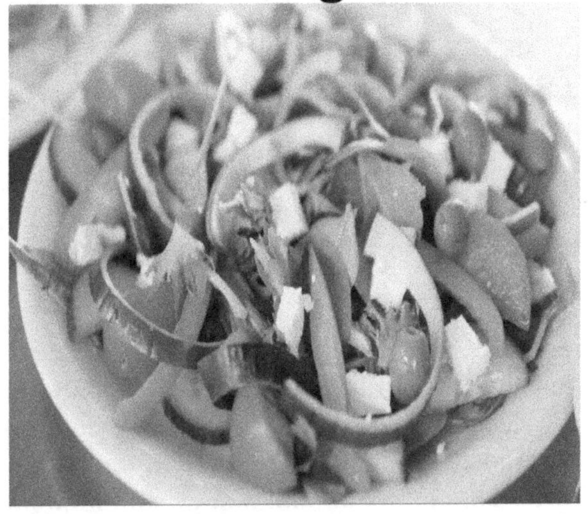

Steven more

Copyright © [2023] by [Steven more]

Table of contents

Introduction

Welcome to "The Complete Plant-Based Cookbook for Beginners," a culinary journey that celebrates the vibrant world of plant-based cooking.

Whether you're a seasoned vegan or just starting to explore the benefits of a plant-centric lifestyle, this cookbook is your compass for delicious and nutritious meals.Embark on a flavorful adventure as we unravel the art of crafting satisfying dishes that showcase the diverse array of plant-based ingredients. From hearty mains to delectable desserts, each recipe is thoughtfully curated to simplify your transition to a plant-based diet. Discover the joy of creating meals that not only nourish your body but also tantalize your taste buds.This cookbook is more than a collection of recipes; it's a guide for those taking their first steps into the plant-based world. Learn essential cooking techniques, understand the nutritional benefits of plant-based ingredients, and master the art of balancing flavors. With easy-to-follow instructions and accessible ingredients, you'll find joy in preparing meals that promote health and well-being.Get ready to embrace a culinary adventure that not only respects the planet but also elevates your kitchen skills.The Complete Plant-Based Cookbook for Beginners" invites you to savor the richness of plant-powered living—one delicious recipe at a time.Chapter one Comprehensive Guide to Plant- Plant-Based Breakfast is not only nutritious but also diverse, offering a plethora of options for those embracing a plant-centric lifestyle. Here's a comprehensive guide to crafting satisfying and nourishing plant-based breakfastst

CHAPTER ONE

Plant-Based Breakfast:

Plant-based breakfasts are not only nutritious but also diverse, offering a plethora of options for those embracing a plant-centric lifestyle. Here's a comprehensive guide to crafting satisfying and nourishing plant-based breakfasts:

1. Foundation

a. Whole Grains:

   oats, Quinoa, and Buckwheat:Use whole grains as a base for breakfast bowls, porridge, or granola, providing complex carbohydrates and fiber.

   variety: Encourage experimenting with different grains to add texture and flavor diversity.

b. Breads and Wraps.

   Whole Grain or Sourdough Bread. Opt for nutrient-dense bread for toasts, sandwiches, or avocado toast.

   Wraps:Consider whole-grain wraps for plant-based breakfast burritos or wraps with various fillings.

2. Protein-Rich Options:

a.Plant-Based Yogurt: Soy, Almond, or Coconut Yogurt: Provide dairy-free yogurt alternatives for parfaits, smoothie bowls, or as a standalone breakfast.

   Probiotics: Highlight the probiotic benefits of plant-based yogurts for gut health.

b.Legumes:

Chickpea Flour Pancakes or Tofu Scramble:Incorporate legumes into breakfast for a protein boost, offering savory and hearty options.

Hummus or Nut Butter:Use as spreads or dips for added protein and flavor.

c. Nuts and Seeds:

Chia Pudding or Overnight Oats: Utilize chia seeds for a pudding consistency or mix with oats for a hearty, nutrient-packed breakfast.

Smoothie Additions: Include nuts, seeds, or nut butters in smoothies for added protein and healthy fats.

3.Fruits and Vegetables:

a. Fresh Fruit:

Berries, Citrus, and Tropical Fruits:Add a burst of flavor, natural sweetness, and a dose of vitamins to breakfast. - Smoothie Bowls:Create vibrant and nutritious bowls with blended fruits as the base.b. Vegetable Additions:

Leafy Greens: Incorporate spinach or kale into smoothies or tofu scrambles for added nutrients.

Avocado:Use for toasts, wraps, or as a topping to provide healthy fats and creaminess.

4. Breakfast Bowls:

a. Açaí or Smoothie Bowls:

Base Options: Use açaí, banana, or other frozen fruits as a base for a thick and refreshing bowl.

Toppings:Include granola, nuts, seeds, and fresh fruit for texture and variety.

b. Grain Bowls:
   Savory or Sweet
Options:Experiment with savory grain
bowls featuring tofu, sautéed
vegetables, and avocado, or sweet
bowls with fruits and nuts.
   Herbs and Spices:Use fresh herbs,
spices, or nutritional yeast for added
flavor.

5. Warm Breakfasts:

a. Porridge and Oatmeal:
   Plant Milk Options:Cook oats with
almond, soy, or coconut milk for a
creamy texture.
   Toppings:Customize with fruits,
nuts, seeds, and a drizzle of maple
syrup or agave.
b. Breakfast Burritos or Tacos:
 Bean Fillings:Fill tortillas with black
beans, sautéed vegetables, avocado,
and salsa for a savory, satisfying
option.
   Tofu Scramble:Use seasoned tofu
as a scramble or filling for breakfast
tacos.
6. Beverages:
a. Plant-Based Milk:
   - Nut, Seed, or Legume-Based
Milks: Choose from almond, coconut,
soy, oat, or pea milk for cereal, coffee,
or as a base for smoothies.
   Homemade Options:Include recipes
for making plant-based milk at home.

Chapter two

Beans and grains

Beans and grains are essential components of plant-based diets, offering a rich array of nutrients and contributing to overall health and well-being. Let's delve into the nutritional benefits, versatility, and sustainable aspects of incorporating beans and grains into plant-based meals.
Nutritional Benefits.
1.Protein:Beans and grains are excellent sources of plant-based protein.They contain essential amino acids, making them valuable alternatives to animal proteins for individuals following a vegetarian or vegan diet.
2. Fiber: Both beans and grains are high in dietary fiber, promoting digestive health and aiding in weight management. Fiber also helps stabilize blood sugar levels, contributing to overall metabolic health.
3. Vitamins and Minerals: These plant-based foods are rich in various vitamins and minerals such as B-vitamins, iron, zinc, magnesium, and potassium, supporting various physiological functions within the body.
Versatility in Cooking:
1. Diverse Culinary Uses: Beans and grains can be prepared in numerous ways, offering a wide range of culinary possibilities. From salads and stews to

burgers and curries, their versatility makes them adaptable to various cultural cuisines.

2. Texture and Flavor:Beans and grains bring unique textures and flavors to dishes. For instance, the nutty taste of quinoa or the creamy texture of lentils can enhance the palatability of plant-based meals.

3. Substitutes in Recipes:They can also serve as substitutes for meat in many recipes. For example, lentils can replace ground meat in tacos, and chickpeas can be used to make plant-based burgers.

Sustainable Impact:

1. Environmental Benefits: Beans and grains have a lower environmental impact compared to animal-based protein sources. They generally require less land, water, and produce fewer greenhouse gas emissions, making them more sustainable choices.

2.Crop Rotation: Growing legumes like beans can improve soil health by fixing nitrogen, benefiting subsequent crops in a rotation. This sustainable agricultural practice contributes to long-term soil fertility.

3. Biodiversity: Including a variety of beans and grains in a plant-based diet promotes biodiversity in agriculture. Diversified cropping systems are more resilient to pests and diseases, reducing the need for synthetic pesticides.

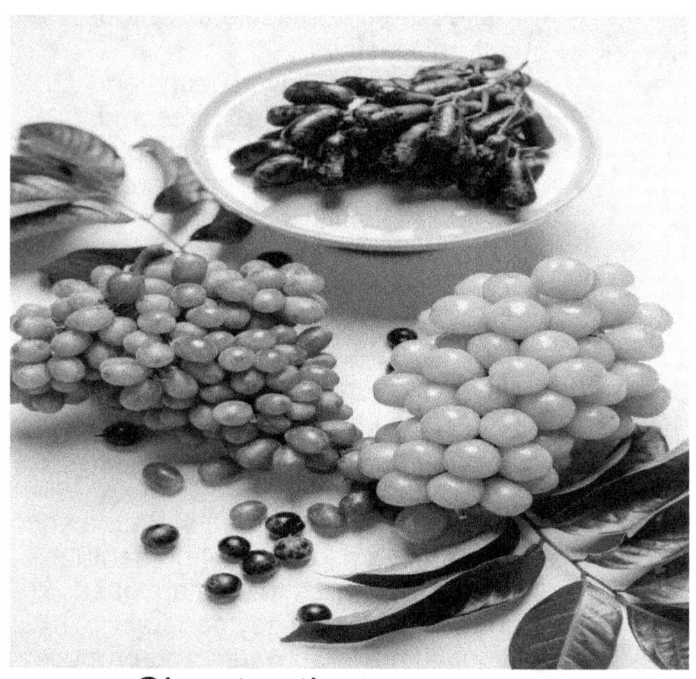

Chapter three
Basics of Plant-Based Foods:

A plant-based diet focuses on consuming whole, minimally processed foods derived from plants. This dietary approach is rich in nutrients, fiber, and antioxidants, offering numerous health benefits. Let's explore the fundamental aspects of plant-based foods:

1:Foundational Plant-Based Food Groups

a. Fruits and Vegetables:

  Variety: Emphasize a diverse range of colors and types to ensure a broad spectrum of vitamins, minerals, and antioxidants.

Fresh and Seasonal:Opt for fresh, seasonal produce to maximize flavor and nutritional content.

b. Whole Grains:

- Examples: Include quinoa, brown rice, oats, barley, and whole wheat products to provide essential carbohydrates, fiber, and various nutrients.

Cooking Techniques: Explore different cooking methods such as boiling, steaming, and baking to prepare grains.

c. Legumes:Sources: Incorporate beans, lentils, chickpeas, and peas for plant-based protein, fiber, and a range of vitamins and minerals.

Canned vs. Dried:Highlight the options of using both canned and dried legumes, with proper preparation techniques.

d. Nuts and Seeds:

Nutrient Density:Include almonds, walnuts, chia seeds, flaxseeds, and more for healthy fats, protein, and omega-3 fatty acids.

Snacking: Showcase their versatility as snacks, toppings, or ingredients in various dishes.

e. Plant-Based Proteins:

Tofu and Tempeh Explore soy based protein sources, providing alternatives to animal proteins.

Plant Based Meat Substitutes:Introduce products made from legumes, grains, or mycoprotein for those transitioning from a meat-based diet.

2. Nutritional Considerations:

a. Protein:

Combining Sources:Emphasize the importance of combining different plant-based protein sources to ensure a well rounded amino acid profile.

Examples: Quinoa, soy products, and legumes are excellent protein sources.

b. Calcium:

Plant Sources:Highlight calcium-rich plant foods like leafy greens (kale, broccoli), fortified plant milk, and tofu.

Absorption: Discuss factors affecting calcium absorption, such as vitamin D and magnesium.

c. Iron:

Plant Iron vs. Animal Iron:Clarify the differences and emphasize the absorption-enhancing role of vitamin C from fruits and vegetables.

Plant Sources: Promote iron-rich foods like lentils, beans, and fortified cereals.

d. Vitamins and Antioxidants:

- Whole Food Sources:Encourage the consumption of a variety of fruits and vegetables for a broad spectrum of vitamins and antioxidants.

- Colorful Plate:Remind individuals that a colorful plate often signifies a nutrient-rich meal.

3. Cooking and Meal Preparation:

a. Cooking Techniques:

Minimally Processed: Emphasize the use of whole, minimally processed ingredients to retain nutritional value.

-Experimentation:Encourage experimentation with different cooking methods to enhance flavors and textures.

b. Meal Planning:

Balanced Meals:Guide individuals in creating balanced meals that include a mix of plant-based protein, carbohydrates, healthy fats, and a variety of vegetables.

Preparation Tips:Provide practical tips for batch cooking and meal prepping to simplify plant-based eating.

4. Sustainability and Environmental Impact:

a. Plant-Based vs. Animal-Based Impact:

Resource Efficiency:Discuss the environmental benefits of plant-based diets, including reduced land use, water consumption, and greenhouse gas emissions.

Biodiversity:Highlight how plant-based agriculture can contribute to biodiversity and sustainable food systems.

b. Seasonal and Local Choices:

Eco-Friendly Practices: Encourage choosing seasonal and locally sourced produce to support sustainable agricultural practices

Reducing Food Waste:Provide tips on minim

Chapter four

Plant-Based Salads:

Salads are a versatile and essential component of a plant-based diet, offering a delightful array of flavors, textures, and nutrients. A plant-based cookbook can showcase the creativity and variety that salads bring to the table. Here's a comprehensive guide:

1. Foundation:

a. Leafy Greens:

Variety: Include a mix of dark, leafy greens such as spinach, kale, arugula, and romaine lettuce for diverse textures and nutrient profiles.

Nutritional Boost: Highlight the rich content of vitamins, minerals, and antioxidants in leafy greens.

b. Colorful Vegetables:

Rainbow Approach:Encourage a colorful mix of vegetables like tomatoes, bell peppers, carrots, cucumbers, and radishes for visual appeal and varied nutrients.

Raw vs. Cooked:Offer options for raw and cooked vegetables to cater to different preferences.

c. Fresh Herbs:

Flavor Enhancement: Introduce herbs like basil, mint, cilantro, and parsley to elevate the overall taste of the salad.

Nutrient Boost:Emphasize the nutritional benefits herbs bring, including anti-inflammatory properties.

2. Protein Sources:

a. Legumes:

Chickpeas, Lentils, and Beans:Incorporate cooked or roasted legumes for plant-based protein, fiber, and a satisfying texture.

Variety: Showcase different legume varieties to diversify nutrient intake.

b. Nuts and Seeds:

Crunch and Nutrients: Include almonds, walnuts, pumpkin seeds, or sunflower seeds for added crunch, healthy fats, and protein.

Toasting:Highlight the flavor enhancement achieved by toasting nuts and seeds.

c. Tofu or Tempeh:

Marination:Provide recipes for marinated and grilled tofu or tempeh to add protein and a savory element to salads.

Texture Variation: Discuss the importance of proper preparation to achieve desired textures.

3. Whole Grains:

a. Quinoa, Farro, or Bulgur:

Cooking Tips:Share techniques for cooking grains to perfection, ensuring they contribute a hearty element to the salad.

Cold vs. Warm:Explore the versatility of using grains in both cold and warm salads.

b. Crispy Ingredients:

Baked Chickpeas or Quinoa Crisps:Introduce crispy elements for texture variation, turning salads into satisfying and substantial meals.

Homemade Croutons: Provide healthier alternatives to traditional croutons, such as whole-grain or sourdough options.

4. Dressings and Vinaigrettes:

a. Homemade Dressings:

Base Ingredients: Emphasize the use of olive oil, balsamic vinegar, citrus, and mustard for creating flavorful, plant-based dressings.

Herbs and Spices:Encourage experimenting with various herbs and spices to tailor dressings to personal preferences.

b. Avocado or Nut-Based Dressings:

Creamy Textures:Introduce avocado or nut-based dressings for a creamy texture without dairy, adding richness to salads.

Healthy Fats: Highlight the benefits of incorporating healthy fats into dressings for better nutrient absorption.

5. Creative Salad Ideas:

a. International Flavors:

Mediterranean, Asian, or Mexican-Inspired Salads:Showcase global influences to add diversity and excitement to plant-based salads.

Fusion Options:Encourage combining ingredients from different cuisines for a unique twist.

b. Fruit Additions:

Berries, Citrus, or Mango:Incorporate fruits for sweetness, acidity, and an extra nutritional boost.

Balance:Emphasize the importance of balancing sweet and savory elements in fruit-infused salads.

6. Serving Suggestions:

a. Presentation:

Layering vs. Tossing: Guide on different ways to present salads, whether layered for aesthetic appeal or tossed for even distribution of flavors.

Edible Bowls:Suggest using large lettuce leaves or bowls made of edible ingredients for a creative presentation.

b. Accompaniments:

Crusty Bread, Hummus, or Guacamole:Recommend complementary side dishes to turn a salad into a complete and satisfying meal.

Pairing Tips: Provide guidance on pairing salads with other plant-based dishes for a well-rounded dining experience.

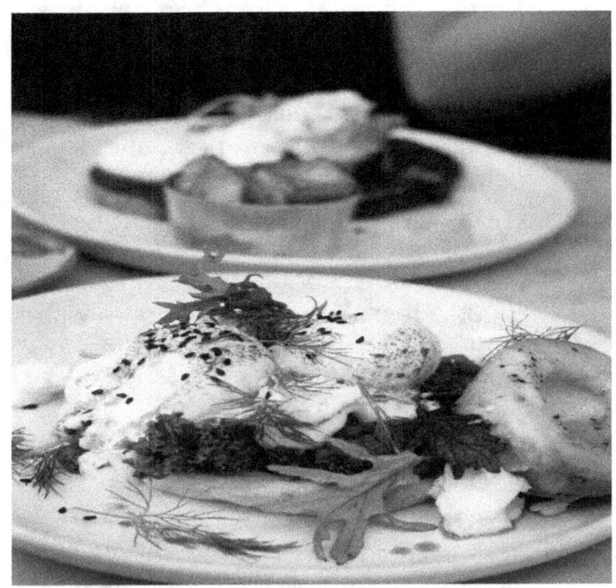

CHAPTER FIVE

Plant-Based Desserts

Plant-based desserts showcase the delightful and indulgent side of a plant-centric diet, proving that sweet treats can be both delicious and nourishing. Here's an extensive guide to crafting a variety of satisfying plant-based desserts:

1. Sweeteners:

a. Natural Sweeteners:

Maple Syrup, Agave Nectar, or Date Syrup:Use these as alternatives to refined sugars to add sweetness to desserts.

Molasses and Coconut Sugar:Explore richer flavors provided by these natural sweeteners.

b. Whole Fruits

Bananas, Dates, and Berries:Incorporate mashed bananas, date paste, or pureed berries to naturally sweeten desserts.

Dried Fruits: Utilize raisins, apricots, or figs for added sweetness and chewiness.

2. Flour Alternatives:

a. Nut and Seed Flours:

Almond, Coconut, or Hazelnut Flour:Substitute traditional flours with these for a nutty flavor and gluten-free options.

Ground Flaxseeds or Chia Seeds:Provide a binding agent and additional nutritional benefits.

b. Whole Grain Flours:

Oat, Spelt, or Whole Wheat Flour:Use whole grains to add fiber and nutrients to desserts.

Quinoa or Buckwheat Flour:Explore gluten-free alternatives with distinct flavors.

3. Plant-Based Fats:

a.Avocado and Nut Butters:

- Avocado Mousse:Create creamy and rich mousses or frostings with ripe avocados.

- Nut Butter Swirls:Add depth and richness by incorporating almond, peanut, or cashew butter.

b. Coconut Products:

Coconut Milk or Cream:Enhance creaminess in desserts like puddings, ice creams, or curds.

- Shredded Coconut or Coconut Oil:Offer texture and flavor variations.

4. Dairy Alternatives:

a. Plant-Based Milk:

Almond, Soy, or Oat Milk:Use in baking, puddings, or custards as substitutes for dairy milk.

Cashew or Macadamia Milk:Add richness to desserts without overpowering flavors.
b. Plant-Based Yogurt:
   Coconut or Almond Yogurt:Incorporate into desserts for a tangy flavor and creamy texture.
   Cashew Cream:Create a versatile base for various sweet dishes.
5. Egg Replacements:
a.Flax Eggs or Chia Eggs:
   Binding Agent: Use these gel-like substitutes to bind ingredients in baked goods.
   Nutritional Boost:Introduce additional fiber and omega-3 fatty acids.
b. Banana or Applesauce:
   Moisture and Binding:Employ mashed bananas or applesauce for moisture and sweetness in desserts.
   Flavor Enhancer:Capitalize on the natural sweetness these ingredients provide.
6. Creative Dessert Ideas:
a. No-Bake Treats:
   Raw Energy Balls or Bars: Combine nuts, seeds, dried fruits, and sweeteners for quick and nutritious snacks.
   Chilled Pies or Cheesecakes:Utilize coconut oil and nut-based crusts for decadent yet no-bake desserts.
b.Frozen Delights:
   Nice Cream: Blend frozen bananas with flavors like vanilla, chocolate, or fruit for a dairy-free ice cream alternative.
   Fruit Sorbets: Puree frozen fruits with a touch of sweetener for refreshing sorbets.
 7. Flavor Enhancements:

a. Spices and Extracts:
   Cinnamon, Nutmeg, or Cardamom:Add warmth and depth to desserts.
   Vanilla, Almond, or Mint Extract:Infuse desserts with aromatic flavors.
b. Citrus Zest and Juices:
   Lemon, Orange, or Lime Zest:Provide a burst of freshness.
   Citrus Juices: Balance sweetness and add brightness to desserts.
8. Decorative Elements:
a. Edible Flowers and Herbs:
   Lavender, Rose Petals, or Mint Leaves:Garnish desserts with these for visual appeal and subtle aromas.
   Microgreens or Berries:Add pops of color and additional nutrients.
b. Chocolate and Cacao:
   Dark Chocolate or Cacao Nibs: Incorporate into desserts for richness and a hint of bitterness.
   Cocoa Powder:Use in baking, hot drinks, or dusted over treats.
 9. Holiday and Special Occasion Desserts
a. Plant-Based Cakes and Cupcakes:
   Layered Cakes:Experiment with different flavors, frostings, and fillings.
   Cupcake Varieties:Create bite-sized treats with diverse flavor options.
b. Pies and Tarts:
   Fruit Pies or Galettes:Feature seasonal fruits for classic desserts.
   Nut-Based Tarts: Explore crusts made with nut flours for added richness.
 10. Allergen-Free Options:
a. Gluten-Free Desserts:

Almond Flour or Chickpea Flour Baking Cater to those with gluten sensitivities.

Quinoa or Rice Flour Treats:Offer alternatives for traditional flour-based recipes.

b. Allergen-Free Substitutes:

Soy Free and Nut Free Options:Provide variations for individuals with specific dietary restrictions.

Seed-Based Alternatives:Explore sunflower seed butter, pumpkin seed butter, or tahini as alternatives

CHAPTER SIX

VEGETABLES AND SIDES

Vegetables and sides play a pivotal role in plant-based cuisine, providing an abundance of flavors, textures, and nutrients. Here's a comprehensive guide to incorporating vegetables and sides into a plant-based diet:

1. Diverse Vegetable Selection

a. Leafy Greens:

Kale, Spinach, Swiss Chard: Rich in vitamins, minerals, and antioxidants, they can be sautéed, steamed, or used raw in salads.

Collard Greens:Ideal for wraps or hearty side dishes when braised.

b. Cruciferous Vegetables:

Broccoli, Cauliflower, Brussels Sprouts:Versatile for roasting, grilling, or stir-frying, providing fiber and cancer-fighting compounds.

Cabbage:Suitable for coleslaw, sauerkraut, or stir-fries.
c. Root Vegetables:
Sweet Potatoes, Carrots, Beets:Roast, mash, or spiralize for diverse textures and natural sweetness.
Radishes and Turnips:Enjoy raw in salads or pickled for added crunch.
d. Allium Vegetables:
Onions, Garlic, Leeks:Fundamental for flavoring various dishes, from soups to stir-fries.
Shallots:Provide a milder, nuanced onion flavor.
e. Colorful Bell Peppers:
Red, Yellow, Green, Orange: Add vibrant colors and a sweet flavor to salads, stir-fries, or stuffed recipes.
2. Starchy Sides:
a. Whole Grains:
Quinoa, Brown Rice, Farro: Serve as a base for various dishes, providing complex carbohydrates.
Barley and Bulgur:Offer nutty flavors and chewy textures.
b. Potatoes and Squashes:
Roasted Potatoes:Season with herbs or spices for a classic side dish.
Butternut or Acorn Squash: Ideal for roasting, pureeing, or stuffing.
c. Legumes as Sides:
Lentils, Chickpeas, or Black Beans:Provide protein and fiber, perfect for salads, stews, or sides.
Edamame or Peas: Add to grain bowls or stir-fries for a protein boost.
3. Savory Side Dishes:
a. Stir-Fried Vegetables:
Colorful Medley:Combine a variety of vegetables in a quick stir-fry with soy sauce or other flavorful sauces.

Sesame Oil and Ginger:Enhance flavors with sesame oil and fresh ginger.

b. Grilled Veggies:

Zucchini, Eggplant, Mushrooms: Grill for smoky flavors and tender textures.

Asparagus or Artichokes: Perfect for grilling or roasting with olive oil and herbs.

c. Cauliflower Rice or Broccoli Rice:

Low Carb Alternatives: Substitute grains with riced cauliflower or broccoli for a lighter option.

Versatile Base:Use as a base for stir-fries or serve as a side dish.

4. Salads and Slaws:

a. Fresh Salads:

Tomato and Cucumber Salad:Simple yet refreshing, perfect for summer.

Mango and Avocado Salad: Combine sweet and creamy elements with a zesty dressing.

b. Coleslaw Variations:

Classic Cabbage Coleslaw:Mix with vegan mayo or vinaigrette for a crunchy side.

Broccoli Slaw:Substitute traditional cabbage with shredded broccoli for added nutrition.

c. Grain and Bean Salads:

Quinoa and Black Bean Salad:Combine grains, beans, and colorful vegetables for a protein-packed dish.

Tabbouleh: A refreshing Middle Eastern salad with bulgur, herbs, and tomatoes.

5. Plant-Based Sauces and Condiments:

a. Hummus and Dips:

Classic Chickpea Hummus: Serve as a dip for veggies or spread on wraps.

Baba Ganoush: Roasted eggplant dip with tahini for a smoky flavor.

b. Guacamole and Salsas:

Avocado Salsa:Combine avocado, tomatoes, and cilantro for a fresh salsa.

Fruit Salsas: Experiment with mango or pineapple salsas for a sweet and spicy twist.

c. Pesto and Herb Sauces:

Basil Pesto:Use on roasted vegetables or as a pasta sauce.

Chimichurri: An Argentinean sauce with parsley, garlic, and vinegar, perfect for grilled veggies.

6. Fermented Foods:

a. Kimchi and Sauerkraut:

Probiotic Rich: Enhance gut health with these fermented options.

Condiment or Side:Serve as a flavorful accompaniment to various dishes.

b. Pickled Vegetables:

Pickled Radishes or Carrots:Add a tangy and crunchy element to sandwiches or grain bowls.

Quick Pickles:Make a variety of quick pickles with cucumbers, onions, or jalapeños.

7. Dressings and Toppings:

a. Vinaigrettes:

Balsamic, Lemon, or Mustard Vinaigrette: Light dressings for salads or roasted veggies.

Tahini Dressing: Creamy and nutty, perfect for grain bowls or roasted roots.

b. Nutritional Yeast and Seeds:

Nutritional Yeast: Adds a cheesy flavor to vegetables or popcorn.
Sunflower or Pumpkin Seeds:Provide crunch and healthy fats as toppings.

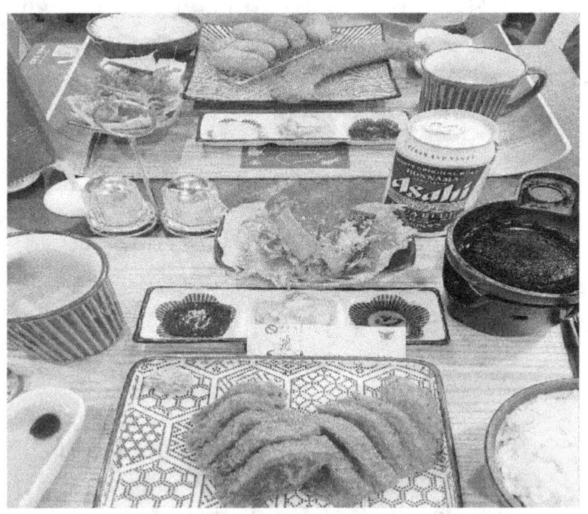

CHAPTER SEVEN

Staples, Sauces, Dips, and Dressings in Plant-Based Cooking:

Plant-based cooking thrives on a foundation of versatile staples, flavorful sauces, and creative dips and dressings. Here's a comprehensive guide to these essential elements that add depth, nutrition, and variety to plant-based cuisine:

1. Plant-Based Staples:

a.Whole Grains:

Quinoa, Brown Rice, Farro:Provide a nutritious base for many dishes, from salads to bowls.

Bulgur and Barley: Add texture and nutty flavors to grain-based recipes.
b. Legumes:
Chickpeas, Lentils, Black Beans:Packed with protein and fiber, versatile for salads, stews, and dips.
Red and Green Lentils:Cook quickly and are excellent for soups and curries.
c. Nuts and Seeds:
Almonds, Walnuts, Chia Seeds:Offer healthy fats, crunch, and a boost of nutrients.
Pumpkin and Sunflower Seeds: Ideal for topping salads or incorporating into granola.
d. Plant-Based Protein Sources:
Tofu and Tempeh: Adaptable to various cooking methods, absorbing flavors and providing a meaty texture.
Seitan and Edamame:Additional protein sources for diverse plant-based meals.
e. Whole Food Sweeteners:
Maple Syrup, Agave Nectar, Date Syrup: Natural alternatives for sweetening desserts and dressings.
Coconut Sugar and Molasses:Add depth and richness to sweet dishes.

a. Tomato-Based Sauces:
Marinara Sauce: A staple for pasta dishes, pizzas, and casseroles.
Tomato Salsa: Fresh and vibrant, perfect for topping various dishes.
b. Creamy Plant-Based Sauces:
Cashew Alfredo Sauce:Rich and creamy, suitable for pasta or vegetable gratins.
Coconut Curry Sauce: Adds depth to curries, stir-fries, or grain bowls.
c. Pesto Varieties:

Classic Basil Pesto: A versatile condiment for pasta, sandwiches, or as a dip.

Spinach or Kale Pesto: Incorporate additional greens for a nutrient boost.

d. Asian-Inspired Sauces:

Teriyaki Sauce: Sweet and savory, perfect for stir-fries and glazing tofu.

Peanut Sauce: Creamy and flavorful, ideal for dipping or drizzling over noodle dishes.

3. Creative Dips:

a. Classic Hummus:

Chickpea Base:Versatile dip for veggies, pita, or as a sandwich spread.

Variations: Experiment with flavors like roasted red pepper or sun-dried tomato hummus.

b. Guacamole and Avocado Dips:

Classic Guacamole: Mashed avocados with tomatoes, onions, and cilantro.

Spicy Avocado Dip:Blend avocados with jalapeños and lime for a zesty kick.

c. Bean Dips:

Black Bean Dip:Spiced black beans blended with herbs for a hearty dip.

White Bean and Rosemary Dip:Creamy and aromatic, suitable for crackers or vegetable sticks.

d. Tahini and Nut-Based Dips:

Tahini Dip: Blend tahini with lemon, garlic, and herbs for a savory dip.

Cashew Cheese Dip: Cashews blended with nutritional yeast for a cheesy flavor.

4. Flavorful Dressings:

a. Balsamic Vinaigrette:

Classic Dressing: Mix balsamic vinegar with olive oil, Dijon mustard, and herbs.

Fruit-Infused Balsamic Dressing:Incorporate berries or citrus for a sweet twist.

b. Lemon Tahini Dressing:

Creamy and Tangy: Blend tahini with lemon juice, garlic, and water for a versatile dressing.

Sesame Ginger Dressing:Asian-inspired with sesame oil, ginger, and soy sauce.

c. Maple-Mustard Dressing:

Sweet and Tangy: Combine maple syrup, Dijon mustard, and apple cider vinegar.

Poppy Seed Dressing: Add poppy seeds for texture and subtle sweetness.

d. Creamy Avocado Dressing:

Avocado Base: Blend ripe avocados with lime, cilantro, and a touch of plant-based yogurt.

Cilantro-Lime Dressing:*Refreshing and herbaceous, perfect for salads or bowls.

5. Condiments and Extras:

a. Nutritional Yeast:

Cheese Substitute:Adds a cheesy flavor to various dishes.

- Popcorn Topping:Sprinkle on popcorn for a savory treat.

b. Pickled Vegetables:

Quick Pickles: Make with cucumbers, radishes, or red onions for a tangy side.

Kimchi: Fermented cabbage, adding a probiotic element to meals.

c. Hot Sauces and Chili Flakes:

Sriracha, Tabasco, or Jalapeño Sauce Elevate flavors with a spicy kick.

Chili Flakes:Add heat to dishes like pizzas or stir-fries.

d. Fresh Herbs and Citrus Zest:

Herb Garnishes: Sprinkle fresh herbs like parsley, basil, or cilantro for a burst of freshness.

Citrus Zest:Grate lemon or orange zest to enhance flavors in salads, sauces, or dressings.

CHAPTER EIGHT

Snacks and Appetizers

Plant-based snacks and appetizers are a delicious way to showcase the diversity and creativity of plant-centric cooking. From light bites to hearty starters, here's a comprehensive guide to crafting flavorful and satisfying plant-based snacks and appetizers:

1. Nutrient-Rich Nibbles:

a. Roasted Chickpeas:

Seasoned Varieties: Toss with spices like cumin, paprika, or nutritional yeast for a crunchy, protein-packed snack.

Sweet Versions:Roast with cinnamon and a touch of maple syrup for a sweet alternative.

b. Mixed Nuts and Seeds:

Trail Mix: Combine almonds, walnuts, pumpkin seeds, and dried fruits for a balanced snack.

Spiced Nuts:Roast with savory or sweet spices for an elevated flavor profile.

c. Edamame:

Steamed or Roasted: Sprinkle with sea salt or chili flakes for a quick and nutritious snack.

Edamame Hummus: Blend with garlic, lemon, and tahini for a protein-rich dip.

2. Creative Plant-Based Dips:

a. Guacamole Variations:

Mango Guacamole:Add diced mango for sweetness and a tropical twist.

Black Bean and Corn Guacamole:Incorporate black beans and corn for added texture.

b. Artichoke and Spinach Dip:

Creamy Base: Use cashews or white beans blended with artichokes and spinach.

- Baked or Chilled:Serve warm or cold with crackers, bread, or vegetable sticks.

c. Beet Hummus:

Vibrant and Nutrient-Packed:Blend chickpeas with roasted beets, garlic, and lemon for a colorful hummus.

Serve with Crudites:Pair with sliced carrots, bell peppers, and cucumber.

3. Fresh and Flavorful Salsas:

a. Classic Salsa Fresca:

Tomato, Onion, and Cilantro: Dice fresh tomatoes, red onion, and cilantro for a traditional salsa.

Peach or Pineapple Salsa:Add a fruity twist with diced peaches or pineapples.

b. Corn and Avocado Salsa:

- Summer Delight: Mix corn kernels, diced avocado, red onion, and lime juice.

Cilantro-Lime Dressing:Drizzle with a zesty cilantro-lime dressing for extra freshness.

c. Mango Salsa:

Sweet and Spicy:Combine diced mango, jalapeño, red onion, and lime juice.

-Serve with Tofu or Plant-Based Tacos:Pair with grilled tofu or plant-based tacos for a tropical flair.

4. Small Bites and Finger Foods:

a. Stuffed Mushrooms:

Quinoa and Spinach Stuffing:Create a flavorful stuffing with quinoa, spinach, and herbs.

Baked or Grilled:Cook until mushrooms are tender for a savory appetizer.

b. Cucumber Rolls:

Thinly Sliced Cucumbers: Fill with hummus, avocado, or plant-based cream cheese.

Colorful Fillings: Add bell peppers, carrots, or sprouts for a burst of color and texture.

c. Stuffed Grape Leaves (Dolma):

Rice and Herb Filling:Wrap grape leaves around a mixture of seasoned rice, pine nuts, and herbs.

Serve with Lemon-Tahini Sauce:Pair with a zesty lemon-tahini dipping sauce.

5. Hearty Plant-Based Dishes:

a. Sweet Potato Bites:

Roasted or Baked:Top sweet potato rounds with guacamole, black beans, or vegan cheese.

Mini Loaded Nachos:Create a plant-based nacho version using sweet potato chips.
b. Vegetable Spring Rolls:
Rice Paper Wrappers: Fill with julienned veggies, tofu, and fresh herbs.
Serve with Peanut Dipping Sauce:Dip in a flavorful peanut sauce for added richness.
c. Stuffed Bell Peppers:
Quinoa or Lentil Filling: Mix with diced tomatoes, black beans, and corn.
Baked or Grilled: Serve as a colorful and satisfying appetizer.
6. Plant-Based Bruschettas:
a. Classic Tomato Bruschetta:
Tomato, Garlic, and Basil:Mix diced tomatoes with garlic, fresh basil, and balsamic glaze.
Serve on Toasted Baguette Slices:Spread on toasted baguette slices for a traditional appetizer.
b. Avocado and White Bean Bruschetta:
Creamy Base:Mash white beans and avocado, season with lemon and herbs.
Top on Crostini:Spread on crostini and garnish with cherry tomatoes.
c. Mushroom and Thyme Bruschetta:
Sautéed Mushrooms:Cook with garlic and thyme for a savory topping.
Add Vegan Cheese:Melt vegan cheese on top for extra richness.
7. International Flavors:
a. Vegan Spring Rolls:
Rice Paper Wrappers: Fill with vermicelli noodles, tofu, mint, and cilantro.

Serve with Peanut Dipping Sauce: Pair with a tangy peanut dipping sauce.

b. Spanakopita Triangles:

Spinach and Vegan Feta Filling:Encase in phyllo pastry for a Greek-inspired appetizer.

Bake until Golden Brown:Achieve a crispy exterior with a golden brown finish.

c. Baba Ganoush Crostini:

Smoky Eggplant Dip: Blend roasted eggplant with tahini, garlic, and lemon juice.

Spread on Crostini or Pita Chips:Serve as a sophisticated dip on crunchy bread or pita chips

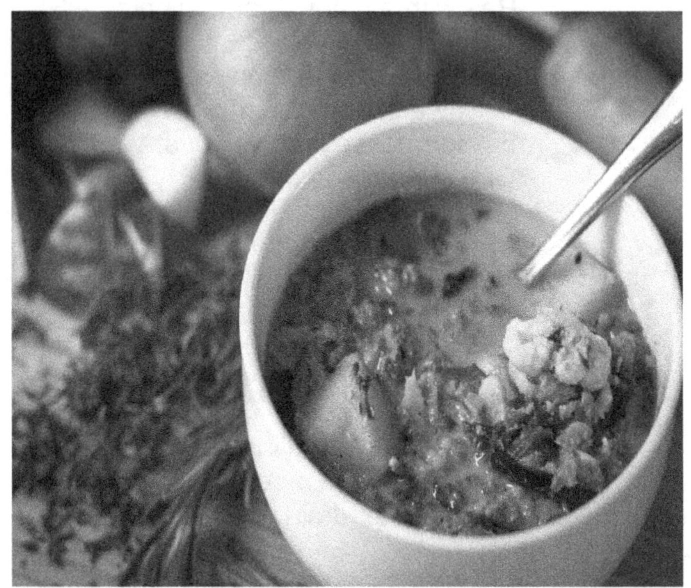

CHAPTER NINE

Stews and Soups

Plant-based stews and soups are nourishing, versatile, and brimming with flavors. Here's a comprehensive guide to understanding and crafting delicious plant-based stews and soups:

Stew:

A stew is a hearty and savory dish where vegetables, legumes, grains, or plant-based proteins are simmered in a flavorful broth until tender.

2. Base Ingredients

Vegetables: Use a variety of vegetables like carrots, potatoes, celery, onions, and bell peppers for depth of flavor.

Legumes:Beans, lentils, or
chickpeas add protein and substance
to the stew.
    Grains:Quinoa, barley, or farro can
be included for texture and additional
nutritional value.
3. Broth or Sauce:
    Vegetable Broth:Provides the
foundation for the stew's flavor.
    Tomato-Based:Tomato sauces or
diced tomatoes contribute richness
and acidity.
    Herbs and Spices: Thyme,
rosemary, bay leaves, cumin, and
paprika add complexity.
4. Protein Sources:
    Plant-Based Proteins Tofu, tempeh,
or seitan be added for a meaty
texture.
    Lentils and Beans: Excellent
sources of protein, fiber, and a variety
of essential nutrients.
5. Cooking Process:
    Slow Simmering:Stews benefit from
slow cooking, allowing flavors to meld
and ingredients to become tender.
    One-Pot Convenience: Ideal for
one-pot cooking, simplifying the
preparation process.
6. Variations:
    Curries:Infuse stews with curry
spices, coconut milk, and aromatics
for a flavorful twist.
    Chili:Create a chili by incorporating
beans, tomatoes, chili powder, and a
mix of spices for a robust and spicy
flavor.
7. Serving Suggestions:
    Grains or Bread:Serve over rice,
quinoa, or with crusty bread for a
complete and satisfying meal.

Garnishes:Fresh herbs, lemon zest, or a drizzle of olive oil can enhance the presentation and taste.

Soups:

1. Definition:

A soup is a liquid dish typically consisting of a broth, vegetables, grains, and sometimes protein, served hot or cold.

2. Base Ingredients:

Broth or Stock:Vegetable broth, mushroom broth, or miso soup base forms the liquid foundation.

- Vegetables: An array of vegetables such as carrots, celery, onions, and leafy greens provides vitamins and minerals.

Grains or Pasta:Rice, noodles, or pasta add substance and texture.

3. Flavor Elements:

Aromatics: Garlic, onions, and herbs like thyme or rosemary add aromatic depth.

Spices:Tailor the spices to your taste, incorporating black pepper, cumin, or turmeric for complexity.

4. Protein Sources:

Tofu or Tempeh:Cubes of tofu or tempeh can be added for protein.

Legumes:Beans or lentils offer a plant-based protein boost.

5. Varieties:

- Minestrone Soup: An Italian vegetable soup featuring tomatoes, beans, and pasta.

Lentil Soup: Protein-rich lentils combined with vegetables and spices.

Gazpacho:A cold Spanish soup made with tomatoes, peppers, onions, cucumbers, and garlic.

6. Cooking Process:

Simmering or Boiling:Soups are typically cooked by simmering or boiling, allowing ingredients to meld and flavors to develop.

Quick Preparation:Some soups, like gazpacho or chilled cucumber soup, require minimal to no cooking.

7. Serving Suggestions:

Bread or Croutons: Accompany with crusty bread, croutons, or crackers for added texture.

Fresh Herbs: Garnish with fresh herbs like parsley or cilantro to enhance freshness.

Vegan Cream: Coconut milk or cashew cream can be used for a creamy texture without dairy.

Key Similarities:

1. Versatility:

Both stews and soups offer endless possibilities for creativity, allowing you to adapt recipes based on seasonal produce and personal preferences.

2.Nutrient Density:

These dishes are inherently rich in plant-based nutrients, providing a wholesome and satisfying eating experience.

3. Customization:

Adapt the recipes by incorporating a variety of vegetables, legumes, grains, and herbs to suit individual tastes.

4. Health Benefits:

Both stews and soups can be crafted to provide a balance of macronutrients, fiber, vitamins, and minerals, contributing to overall well-being.

Conclusion

A plant-based cookbook for beginners is an invaluable resource, offering a diverse array of delicious and nutritious recipes centered around plant-derived ingredients. These cookbooks typically provide comprehensive guidance, making it easy for individuals transitioning to a plant-based lifestyle. From simple breakfast ideas to satisfying main courses and creative desserts, these cookbooks cater to various tastes and preferences.

The extensive variety of recipes ensures that beginners can explore a range of flavors and textures, helping them discover the versatility of plant-based ingredients. Additionally, these cookbooks often include essential information on the nutritional benefits of plant-based eating, aiding beginners in understanding how to achieve a balanced and wholesome diet.

The step-by-step instructions and beginner-friendly tips make the cooking process approachable, even for those with limited culinary experience. Moreover, plant-based cookbooks frequently emphasize the use of readily available ingredients, making it convenient for beginners to incorporate these recipes into their daily lives without the need for complex or hard-to-find items.